50 ways to
take the junk
out of junk food

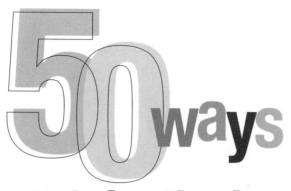

50 ways

to **take the junk out of** junk **food**

**Quick and
Nutritious
Treats
to Make
with
Your Kids**

Julie Whittingham

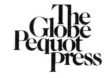

The
Globe
Pequot
Press

GUILFORD, CONNECTICUT

Text design: Nancy Freeborn

Library of Congress Cataloging-in-Publication Data
Whittingham, Julie.
    50 ways to take the junk out of junk food : quick and nutritious treats to make with your kids / Julie Whittingham.
        p. cm.
    Includes index.
    ISBN 0-7627-2869-8
    1. Snack foods. 2. Quick and easy cookery. 3. Low-fat diet—Recipes. 4. Sugar-free diet—Recipes. I. Title: Fifty ways to take the junk out of junk food. II. Title.

TX740.W475 2003
641.5'3—DC22
                        2003049325

Manufactured in the United States of America
First Edition/First Printing

To Rick, Todd, Justen, Michael, and Jamie
Craig, Doug, Steve, and Connie

For the inspiration to create healthy food and
share it with everyone who reads this book.

For letting me be wife and mother to the most
important people in my life.

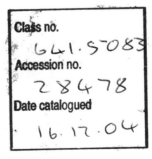

contents

acknowledgments

Special thanks to my best friend, Rhonda, and my mother, Mary, who encouraged me and had the faith in my passion for the pursuit of healthy children. Grateful thanks to my Sunday School class of great kids, who were brave enough to trust my cooking skills, to test my recipes, and to give suggestions on what kids love to eat. Heartfelt thanks to my husband, Rick, who is my soul mate, greatest supporter, and inspiration for writing this book. He reminds me, by his example, to salute the kid in my heart every day. Final thanks to my grandmother, Lucille, who was my hero and is now the angel on my shoulder who helped me write this book.

introduction

Some of my fondest memories of childhood are of the times spent watching my beloved grandmother, Lucille, bake cookies, candies, and other scrumptious treats for my brother, sister, and me to enjoy. To this day, I can't think of my grandmother's desserts without remembering all the wonderful smells that permeated from her kitchen while she was making them.

In the old days this kind of sugary, fat-filled, starchy food meant love, comfort, and security. Grandmothers and mothers were merely trying to pass down the recipes that helped shape their most loving memories as children.

I tried to re-create those special moments with Grandma by making those recipes in my own kitchen with my three little boys. I thought that I was being a good mother by baking cakes, pies, cookies, and candies every week for my family to relish. Did they enjoy them? Absolutely! Did they suffer from tummy aches, mood swings, and allergies? You bet!

I admit that I'm a slow learner, but I really had no idea that on a regular basis I was serving my children "junk food" on a platter.

As my children grew, I began to read books on healthy eating habits that eventually led me to attain a bachelor's degree in nutrition. The more I've learned, the more convinced I've become that the time is now to begin a new tradition of healthy foods and snack treats that will help wipe out the health challenges facing the children of this fast-food society.

Did you know that children can become malnourished from too much refined sugar, white flour, and hydrogenated fats (the little culprits responsible for helping form sticky plaque in our arteries)? These potentially high-risk foods lay the foundation for heart attacks, strokes, and cancer in the adult years. Complications from childhood obesity can include high blood pressure, diabetes, and hormone disorders. The same rich foods that make kids fat may also result in skin problems, enlarged tonsils, ear infections, sinusitis, asthma, tooth decay, and countless digestive problems. Many children become hyperactive and have trouble concentrating after eating sugar and chemically altered foods. Fortunately, doctors are now finding that many forms of physical and mental disorders improve when dietary changes are made.

Our bodies metabolize sugar as sugar no matter what form it comes in, so it must be used wisely and moderately. Honey, molasses, and pure maple syrup are wiser choices because they contain trace minerals and tend to be less likely to disturb blood sugar levels and energy cycles than refined sugar. Raw honey, however, should never be given to children under one year of age.

Nutritionists are now recognizing that refined carbohydrates found in white flour convert very rapidly to blood sugar levels that put stress on the pancreas if eaten frequently. This stress is what can lead to Type II diabetes.

Do not be misled by "no cholesterol" labels on containers of vegetable oils, chocolates, shortenings, margarines, and even peanut butter. They may not contain cholesterol, but they do have hydrogenated fats that can cause our bodies to produce excessive amounts of choles-terol. Moderate amounts of unsweetened or semisweet chocolate or even carob mixed with honey can go a long way toward satisfying that sweet tooth with less stress on the body than a milk chocolate candy bar. Low-fat forms of peanut butter and margarine are better alterna-tives to the higher-fat versions. You may even want to visit your local health food store to experience the mouth-watering taste of natural peanut butter ground with no hydrogenated fats. Of course, children who have allergies to peanuts should never eat any of the peanut or peanut butter recipes.

This easy-to-read book may help prevent or improve any health challenge, but it is not a diet book meant to cure any disease. It is important to note that not all ingredients are for everybody. I encourage you to find substitutes for ingredients that may cause an allergy or food sensitivity. And remember, less is better, especially when eating nuts or dried fruits, to prevent unnecessary tummy aches or diarrhea.

50 Ways to Take the Junk out of Junk Food takes a warmhearted approach to helping children understand the effect their food choices have on their health and well-being. They will be encouraged to realize the power they have to influence their health as they establish lifelong patterns of smart dietary choices. They will have the memorable experi-ence of creating with their favorite grown-ups homemade snacks that are healthier, fun, and delicious options to store-bought candies, cup-cakes, and crackers.

I like to think of this book not as the perfect solution to our chil-dren's fat and sugar addictions but as a book that takes a bold step toward offering wise alternatives to the foods kids love most. While these 50 delicious recipes were inspired by my grandmother's kitchen, they have a few important changes. They are low-fat, natural treats with no added sugar. Most important, they taste great! Kids can participate in the preparation of every simple recipe, many of which take only fifteen minutes to make. Best of all, you will be creating loving memories with your children that will last them a lifetime, only to be shared again with their children in years to come.

I am donating a percentage of the gross proceeds from the sale of each book to the Foster Parents Association.

tips for cooking with kids

This book includes basic techniques and simple recipes for preparing desserts that are nutritious and fun for kids to create. The recipes invite kids' creativity to run free. The two of you can personalize them to your own specific tastes.

- For the sweetest or tartest of fruits, be sure to choose produce that is in season. Better yet, let your little one accompany you to the super-market to help pick out the ingredients the two of you will be using.

- Fruit juices make tasty sauces. Like honey and pure maple syrup, fruit juices are natural sweeteners that easily replace sugar.

- Small amounts of nuts and seeds add texture and protein to many dishes. They are very flavorful but they do contain fat, so a little goes a long way.

- When buying packaged and canned items, always read labels care-fully. Shop together to choose products lowest in fat. Always use pure vanilla extract rather than imitation vanilla, because imitation vanilla is mostly artificial flavorings made with chemicals that often have a harsh quality and can leave a bitter aftertaste. Pure 100 percent maple syrup is a must. The extra expense is well worth the rich taste and natural sweeteners.

- The three P's of cooking with kids can be taught as well as learned by big and little people, but they must be practiced as a guideline for kitchen etiquette to be successful. *Praise* for trying something new; *patience* to work together as a team; and the *persistence* to keep trying so that both of you can enjoy the rewards together.

- Always read the entire recipe with your little one before you begin cooking. It's fun when he or she can read it to you. That way you both will have an idea of what to look forward to and there won't be any surprises.

- Lay out all the ingredients and cooking utensils and equipment before you begin. Let your child organize each ingredient in the order you will be using them so that everything will be close at hand.

- Don't be afraid to substitute an ingredient if you don't care for a particular food item or one of you has a food sensitivity or allergy to the ingredient.

- All young children love a tea party. Why not create your own version? It doesn't matter how you choose to celebrate as long as you remember that the preparation and the sharing of these healthy foods together form memories that last a lifetime. Have fun!

best baked goodies

There's nothing so comforting as that first bite of a warm muffin, cake, or cookie, especially on a rainy day or winter night. These classic baked goodies taste just like they came out of your grandmother's oven. But you'll know you made them the healthy way.

maple cake

Pure maple syrup gives this tasty cake a much richer taste than the artificial stuff that is mostly flavorings made with chemicals, which can leave a bitter aftertaste. The canola oil is a smart alternative to the shortenings my grandmother used, because it bakes up lighter and is cholesterol-free.

3 cups whole wheat flour

¼ teaspoon salt

1 tablespoon baking powder

1 teaspoon ground cinnamon

1 cup pure maple syrup

½ cup canola oil

2 eggs, beaten

1 teaspoon vanilla extract

1 cup low-fat milk

1. Preheat oven to 350°F.
2. Oil and flour a 9-inch round or square or bundt cake pan.
3. In a large bowl, sift together the flour, salt, baking powder, and cinnamon.
4. In another bowl, beat together the maple syrup and canola oil. Stir the eggs, vanilla, and milk into the maple syrup mixture.
5. Stir the wet ingredients into the dry ingredients.
6. Pour the batter into the baking pan. Bake until a cake tester or toothpick inserted in the center comes out clean, 40 to 45 minutes.
7. Cool slightly on a rack before turning out to cool completely. Tastes great with Mama's Whipped Cream (page 57).

Makes one 9-inch round, square, or bundt cake

honey nut corn

Remember how much fun it was to dig into a box of Cracker Jack? Here's a low-calorie treat that kids will love to make with you while you delight in new tastes and old memories.

7 cups air-popped corn
Salt to taste
½ cup peanuts
2 tablespoons honey
3 tablespoons light margarine
½ teaspoon ground cinnamon

1. Preheat oven to 350°F.
2. Put popcorn into a large bowl and flavor it with salt. Mix in peanuts.
3. Put honey, margarine, and cinnamon into a microwave-safe container and cook it on high for 30 seconds.
4. Pour honey mixture over salted popcorn and peanuts. Stir to coat well.
5. Spread popcorn evenly in a lightly oiled jellyroll pan or large sheet pan. Bake 12 to 14 minutes. Stir once while cooking.
6. Let cool 15 minutes before eating or storing in an airtight container.

Serves 4

banana graham squares

Fun to make and heaven to eat. The low-fat graham crackers, light cream cheese, and light margarine are all ways to cut down on calories and fat. These squares are great served with sliced banana and a few chopped walnuts on top and drizzled with a tablespoon of honey.

28 squares low-fat honey graham crackers

⅓ cup light margarine, melted

½ teaspoon ground cinnamon

3 8-ounce packages light cream cheese, softened

¾ cup honey

1 teaspoon vanilla extract

3 eggs

½ cup mashed bananas

1. Preheat oven to 350ºF.
2. Crush graham crackers until they make fine crumbs. Measure; there should be about 2 cups of finely crushed crumbs.
3. Mix the graham cracker crumbs with the melted margarine and cinnamon. Press onto bottom of 13x9x2-inch baking pan.
4. Put cream cheese, honey, vanilla, eggs, and mashed bananas in a large mixing bowl. Combine until well blended with an electric mixer set on medium speed. Pour into the graham cracker crust.
5. Bake for 45 to 50 minutes or until the center is almost set. Remove from oven to cool, then refrigerate for 3 hours.

Serves 18

grandma's favorite apple crisp

This is so good! Grandma used fresh Delicious apples to add an extra bit of sweetness to this dish, and I agree that they are the best apples for this special treat. I'm sure she would forgive me for substituting whole wheat flour, light margarine, granola, and honey in this healthy version of her time-honored dessert.

4 cups peeled and chopped Delicious apples
2 tablespoons whole wheat flour
1 tablespoon ground cinnamon
2 tablespoons light margarine
2 cups granola
1 cup honey

1. Preheat oven to 375°F.
2. Lightly grease a 9-inch cake pan.
3. Place apple pieces in large mixing bowl.
4. Combine flour, cinnamon, and margarine in a separate bowl until mixture is crumbly. Pour over apples and mix together.
5. Add granola and honey to apples and mix well. Bake, uncovered, for 45 minutes, making sure to stir occasionally.
6. Remove from oven and let cool 30 minutes before serving.

Serves 8

cinnamon honey buns

Want a really fast and easy treat? You can have a warm and hearty sweet roll in minutes without having to bring out the rolling pin.

1 pan of 6 wheat buns or rolls ready to brown
   in the oven
3 tablespoons chopped walnuts
¼ teaspoon ground cinnamon
⅓ cup honey

1. Follow the directions on the package for browning the buns.
2. Mix walnuts, cinnamon, and honey.
3. Two minutes before the buns are ready, remove the pan from the oven and brush the honey-nut mixture over them. Return pan to oven for 2 minutes.

Makes 6 buns

bread pudding

This is another of my family's favorites. The addition of honey instead of white sugar is a bit easier on our sugar levels; but like white sugar, a little goes a long way.

2½ slices wheat bread

4 eggs

2 cups low-fat milk

⅓ cup honey

½ teaspoon ground cinnamon

½ teaspoon vanilla extract

¼ teaspoon salt

½ cup raisins

¼ cup honey

1. Lightly toast the bread to dry it out, then cut it into 1-inch cubes. Measure out 2½ cups cubes.
2. Preheat oven to 325°F.
3. Lightly oil an 8x1½-inch round baking dish. Place bread cubes in dish. Sprinkle with raisins.
4. Beat together eggs, milk, ⅓ cup honey, cinnamon, vanilla, and salt.
5. Pour egg mixture over bread cubes. Bake 40 to 45 minutes or until a knife inserted near the center comes out clean.
6. Cool slightly and drizzle with ¼ cup honey before serving.

Serves 6

peach enchiladas

Olé for enchilada desserts that are sweet and saucy. The natural flavors of the ingredients in this recipe blend to make a filling treat that has a wonderfully soft texture. Make sure to use very ripe peaches. Light cream cheese tastes just as good as the fat version and is so much better for keeping our kids fit.

4 ripe peaches
1½ cups orange juice
2 tablespoons honey
1 tablespoon pure maple syrup
¾ cup raisins
4 tablespoons light cream cheese
4 wheat tortillas
½ teaspoon ground cinnamon

1. Preheat oven to 350°F.
2. Peel peaches. Cut into cubes or small pieces. Mash with a fork in a mixing bowl.
3. Combine mashed peaches with orange juice, honey, maple syrup, and raisins.
4. Spread 1 tablespoon of cream cheese on each tortilla.
5. Measure 4 tablespoons of the peach mixture and set aside. Now divide the rest of the peach mixture among the 4 tortillas. Spread it out evenly.
6. Roll up each tortilla and place in 8-inch square baking pan. Top each tortilla with a tablespoonful of the remaining peach mixture. Top with cinnamon.
7. Bake, covered, for 20 minutes. Serve warm.

Serves 4

baked apples

Remember what your mother said about eating an apple a day? It's true! Apples provide fiber for keeping cholesterol levels in check and are loaded with vitamins and antioxidants that help keep our bodies healthy and free from disease. This is a terrific way to get your kids interested in eating more servings of fruit, and it's delicious served with nonfat frozen yogurt.

6 large Delicious apples, cored
½ cup raisins
½ teaspoon ground cinnamon
1 cup pure maple syrup
½ teaspoon vanilla extract
½ teaspoon ground cinnamon
½ teaspoon ground nutmeg
6 tablespoons light margarine

1. Preheat oven to 350ºF. Place the apples in a baking dish.
2. Mix raisins with cinnamon. Stuff mixture into apples.
3. Combine maple syrup, vanilla, cinnamon, and nutmeg.
4. Dot the top of each apple with 1 tablespoon margarine and pour the maple syrup mixture over the top.
5. Bake, uncovered, for about 45 minutes or until apples are tender, basting every 15 minutes.

Serves 6

maple chips

These chips are so much better for you than a bag of chips or cookies. They satisfy any sweet tooth and are so easy to prepare. Instead of making strips, you can get out your cookie cutters and make funny shapes with your children. Don't be afraid to use your imagination.

> 2 slices whole wheat bread
> 1 tablespoon light margarine
> 2 tablespoons pure maple syrup
> ½ teaspoon ground cinnamon

1. Preheat oven to 375°F.
2. Spread ½ tablespoon margarine on each piece of bread.
3. Spread 1 tablespoon maple syrup and ¼ teaspoon cinnamon on each piece of bread.
4. Place the 2 slices of bread together and cut off crusts. Place between 2 pieces of waxed paper and use a rolling pin to carefully flatten the bread.
5. Cut the bread into 6 strips, then cut the strips in half. Spread evenly on cookie sheet and bake for 15 minutes. Remove from oven and cool before serving.

Makes 12 pieces

gingerbread cupcakes

You will love the aroma your kitchen sends out while baking these no-sugar, no-shortening, no-white-flour treats. You will also enjoy knowing that by choosing to cook with these ingredients you are helping prevent common childhood disorders such as obesity, tooth decay, allergies, digestive problems, and the onset of Type II diabetes.

2 cups whole wheat pastry flour
1 teaspoon baking soda
1 teaspoon ground ginger
1 teaspoon ground cinnamon
1/2 teaspoon ground cloves
1/2 teaspoon ground nutmeg
1/8 teaspoon allspice
1/2 cup canola oil
1 1/2 cups pure maple syrup
1/2 cup molasses
2 eggs, separated
1/2 cup plain yogurt

1. Preheat oven to 350°F. Set paper baking cups in a 12-cup muffin tin.
2. In a large bowl, mix together the flour, baking soda, ginger, cinnamon, cloves, nutmeg, and allspice.
3. In another bowl, beat together the oil, maple syrup, and molasses.
4. In a small bowl, lightly beat the egg yolks. Add them to the wet ingredients. Stir in the yogurt.
5. Combine the flour mixture with the wet ingredients, stirring well.
6. In another large bowl, beat the egg whites until stiff. Fold them into the batter.
7. Pour the batter into the muffin tin. Bake 25 to 30 minutes or until a toothpick or cake tester inserted into the center comes out clean.
8. Cool cupcakes in the muffin tin, set on a rack. Spread with Lemon Cream-Cheese Sauce (page 59) if desired.

Makes 12 cupcakes

yummy apple cookies

Yummy is the key word here. I love the idea of teaching children how to cook responsibly for themselves while enjoying the benefits of their wise food choices. They will love these cookies and will cherish their memories of baking them with their favorite grown-up.

1 cup whole wheat pastry flour
1 teaspoon baking powder
¼ teaspoon salt
1 teaspoon ground cinnamon
1 cup quick-cooking rolled oats
½ cup chopped toasted walnuts
⅓ cup raisins
1 peeled and minced Delicious apple
1 cup pure maple syrup
¼ cup canola oil
½ teaspoon vanilla extract
1 egg

1. Preheat oven to 375ºF. Oil a cookie sheet.

2. In a large bowl, combine the flour, baking powder, salt, cinnamon, and oats. Stir in the nuts, raisins, and apple.

3. In a separate bowl, whisk together the maple syrup, oil, vanilla, and egg. Stir into the flour mixture until well blended.

4. Using a wet teaspoon to prevent sticking, drop batter onto the prepared cookie sheet. Flatten the cookies with your fingers to ½ inch thick.

5. Bake until golden brown, 10 to 12 minutes. Cool 2 minutes on the cookie sheet, and then transfer to a rack to cool completely.

Makes 3 dozen cookies

spicy oat muffins

A delicious treat to start out the day when there is no time to make a bowl of steaming oatmeal. Why not make these with your child the night before and heat them up the next morning for a hearty breakfast warm-up? Raisins, yogurt, and oatmeal sound like a perfect combination to me, especially with a glass of milk or juice.

2 tablespoons molasses

$\frac{1}{2}$ cup honey

2 eggs

$\frac{1}{4}$ cup low-fat plain yogurt

$\frac{1}{4}$ cup low-fat milk

$\frac{1}{2}$ cup old-fashioned oats

1 cup whole wheat flour

$1\frac{1}{2}$ teaspoons baking powder

$1\frac{1}{2}$ teaspoons ground ginger

1 teaspoon ground cloves

$\frac{1}{2}$ teaspoon ground cinnamon

$\frac{1}{4}$ cup chopped walnuts

$\frac{1}{4}$ cup raisins

1. Preheat oven to 350°F. Rub oil into a 12-cup muffin tin.
2. Combine molasses and honey in microwave-safe bowl and heat on high for 30 seconds. Set aside.
3. Whisk eggs, yogurt, and milk together until blended. Stir in cooled molasses and honey mixture.
4. Add the oats, flour, baking powder, and all the spices. Stir well.
5. Fold in walnuts and raisins.
6. Pour batter into the muffin tin. Bake for 15 to 20 minutes. Cool 30 minutes before serving.

Makes 12 muffins

macaroon muffins

Coconut gives a flavorful and different texture to these muffins, making them a bit richer in taste than the typical muffin. Kids love them and probably don't even realize that they are eating something that is good for them.

1½ cups whole wheat flour

1 cup old-fashioned oats

2 teaspoons baking powder

1 teaspoon ground cinnamon

1 cup low-fat milk

1 egg

¼ cup canola oil

½ teaspoon vanilla extract

½ cup honey

½ cup raisins

1 cup shredded coconut

1. Preheat oven to 375°F. Lightly grease a 12-cup muffin tin.
2. Mix together the flour, oats, baking powder, and cinnamon.
3. In a separate bowl, whisk together the milk, egg, oil, vanilla, and honey. Add to the dry ingredients and stir until smooth.
4. Fold in raisins and coconut.
5. Pour batter into the greased muffin cups. Bake 20 to 25 minutes. Serve warm.

Serves 12

strawberry jam bars

No artificial ingredients and all-natural flavors enhance the goodness of these bars. Bet you can't eat just one.

2 cups quick-cooking rolled oats
1 cup whole wheat flour
1 teaspoon baking powder
1 teaspoon ground cinnamon
½ teaspoon ground ginger
⅛ teaspoon ground nutmeg
¼ teaspoon salt
½ cup pure maple syrup
½ cup canola oil
1 teaspoon vanilla extract
1 10-ounce jar no-sugar-added strawberry jam

1. Preheat oven to 350°F. Oil a 9x9-inch baking pan.
2. In a large bowl, combine the oats, flour, baking powder, and spices.
3. In another bowl, beat together the maple syrup, canola oil, and vanilla.
4. Stir the wet mixture into the dry, mixing until blended.
5. Press half the mixture into the prepared baking pan. Gently spread the jam on top. Sprinkle the remaining crust mixture over the jam, making sure the dough gets into the corners of the pan. Gently pat the topping smooth.
6. Bake until golden brown, about 45 minutes. Cool completely before cutting into bars.

Makes about 12 bars

Coolest Candies

Everyone loves candy, but most of the candy
we buy has nothing nutritional to offer. Give
your children a better choice with these five
melt-in-your-mouth candies.

peanut butter oat balls

Peanut butter is a favorite for people of all ages, but low-fat peanut butter is better for you. Combine it with honey, raisins, and any unsweetened toasted cereal, and now you've got a winner with a crunchy, melt-in-your-mouth taste. It's full of protein, too!

1 cup low-fat chunky peanut butter
1 tablespoon honey
½ cup raisins
2 cups unsweetened toasted oat cereal

1. Mix peanut butter, honey, and raisins until thoroughly combined.
2. Shape into teaspoon-size balls.
3. Pour the toasted oats onto a plate. Roll the balls in the oats until completely covered.
4. Place the balls on a plate covered with waxed paper. Chill in refrigerator for about 1 hour before serving.

Makes about 24 balls

crazy crispy balls

Who doesn't like Rice Krispie squares? Remove the marshmallows and butter and replace them with honey and light margarine and you have yourself a close version of an all-time favorite.

1 stick light margarine

1 cup honey

1/8 teaspoon salt

1/2 cup raisins

3 cups crispy rice cereal

1 cup whole nuts

1 teaspoon vanilla extract

1. Mix together margarine, honey, salt, and raisins in a saucepan. Simmer for 8 minutes.

2. Remove from heat. Stir in cereal, nuts, and vanilla.

3. Set aside to cool. When cool enough to handle, form into small balls for serving. Store any leftovers in the refrigerator.

Makes 24

sunflower seed honey kisses

These kisses couldn't be easier to make. You will have fun preparing them with your child and more fun sharing them with friends. Honey is a little easier on our sugar levels, but like white sugar it needs to be eaten in moderation because too much of any type of sugar can lead to disorders such as diabetes. Remember, no raw honey for babies under one year of age.

> 12 half-teaspoons creamy clover honey
> 1 cup salted sunflower seeds

1. Shape creamy honey into 12 balls. (Spoons used to make melon balls are useful here, but they are not required.) Lightly wet spoon with water to prevent sticking.
2. Roll each ball in sunflower seeds.
3. Place on waxed paper and refrigerate for 1 hour.

Makes 12 candies

pea-nutty squares

Your youngster is sure to make a hit with these squares at a party or sleep-over. The two of you can prepare these squares ahead of time and pull them out of the refrigerator for a festive surprise.

1 square (1 ounce) semisweet chocolate

½ cup honey

½ cup creamy low-fat peanut butter

1 cup roasted soybeans or dry roasted peanuts

1 cup raisins

1 cup flaked coconut

½ cup crushed cornflakes

1. Melt chocolate in microwave oven in a microwave-safe dish for 1 minute.

2. Put honey and peanut butter into another microwave-safe dish. Heat for 1 minute on high in a microwave oven. Stir to combine.

3. Stir melted chocolate into melted honey and peanut butter until smooth.

4. Stir in soybeans or peanuts, raisins, and coconut.

5. Line a 9x5x3-inch loaf pan with waxed paper. Press mixture evenly into pan.

6. Sprinkle with cornflakes. Cover and chill until firm.

7. Cut into squares. Store, covered, in refrigerator.

Makes 24 pieces

fun dates

Any dried fruit is like candy to me. It is full of good things like iron to make strong bones and red blood cells. Moderation, however, is the key to eating these date candies to prevent raising sugar levels too high or causing stomach upsets. Carob is a good alternative to chocolate because it is gentler on the digestive tract.

12 large dates
12 almonds
12 teaspoons light cream cheese
12 teaspoons semisweet chocolate chips or
    carob chips

1. Slice each date in half, being sure to remove the pit.
2. Place one almond on one side of each date half and 1 teaspoon cream cheese on the other half.
3. Sprinkle 1 teaspoon of chips on the cream cheese.
4. Press halves together and chill in refrigerator for 1 hour.

Makes 12 date candies

delightful drinks

It's too easy to reach for bottled drinks or sodas when your children are thirsty. Here are four beverages that not only are better for them but also are like a refreshing dessert in a glass.

berry good lemonade

My second name for this lemonade is Antioxidant Ade, because it is jam-packed with vitamins that help protect against colds, flu, and infections. It's fun to drink because of the berry surprises at the bottom of the glass.

4 large juicy lemons

½ cup or more honey

3½ cups water

1 cup raspberries, boysenberries, mulberries, blackberries, or strawberries

1. Squeeze lemons into a large pitcher. Remove any seeds. Slowly stir in the honey. Taste, and add more honey as needed.
2. When thoroughly mixed, add water and berries. Pour lemonade into glasses that are half full of ice.

Serves 6

honey-kissed hot chocolate

Why settle for an envelope of sickeningly sweet and artificially flavored cocoa when you can easily make it from scratch? The kids will enjoy the process of making a cup of hot chocolate that tastes every bit as good as a powdered mix. I like it better!

⅓ cup water

⅛ teaspoon salt

4 tablespoons unsweetened cocoa powder

4 tablespoons honey

3 cups low-fat milk

1. Combine water, salt, and cocoa powder in a medium-size saucepan. Place it over medium heat and bring it to a simmer.
2. Stir for 2 minutes until smooth.
3. Add honey and milk. Simmer, stirring for 1 minute, then remove from heat and serve. Do not let it boil.

Serves 4

Icy Grape Drink

A delightfully colorful drink that packs a real flavor punch. Fun to drink, but beware of the purple mustache it creates with every sip.

2 cups prepared purple grape juice

12 purple grapes

1 25-ounce bottle sparkling purple grape juice

1. Pour grape juice into a 12-cube ice tray. Drop a grape in the middle of each cube. Put ice tray in freezer and leave it until the cubes are frozen.
2. Remove cubes from ice tray and put 3 cubes in each of 4 glasses. Pour sparkling grape juice over ice cubes and serve with a straw.

Makes 4 glasses

Banana Strawberry Shake

Making a shake together is always fun and a perfect opportunity to talk about each ingredient you put in the blender. Why not celebrate by making a toast to your good health?

2 ripe bananas, sliced

²/₃ cup sliced strawberries

1 cup frozen vanilla nonfat yogurt

1 cup orange juice

2 whole strawberries

1. Place bananas, sliced strawberries, yogurt, and orange juice in a blender. Blend just until mixed so that the mixture is thick and creamy.

2. Pour into malt glasses or tall glasses and top each glass with a whole strawberry.

Serves 2

fabulous fruits

Fruits and their juices can be a good source of extra water and quick energy on a hot or active day. They are also high in vitamin C, calcium, iron, phosphorus, magnesium, chromium, and some B-complex vitamins—great building blocks for bones, blood, and nervous systems. Let your imagination be your guide in creating the juicy dishes in this chapter.

fruity graham parfait

How about graham crackers and milk with your favorite fruit? Better yet, serve it all up in a fancy parfait glass and have yourselves a party.

Graham cracker crumbs
Fresh fruit, sliced
Mama's Whipped Cream (page 57)

1. Mix together equal amounts of graham cracker crumbs and your favorite sliced fruit.
2. Pour into parfait glasses and top with Mama's Whipped Cream. Serve immediately.

coolest pear sundae

I remember making chocolate sundaes with Grandma when I was a little girl. They were special times because we were simply celebrating being together. You can do that too, but try this healthier version of that all-time-favorite dessert.

1 ripe pear, cored, peeled, and quartered
¼ cup slivered blanched almonds
½ cup Honey Chocolate Sauce (page 56)

1. Place 2 pear pieces in each dessert dish. Sprinkle pears with almonds.
2. Pour ¼ cup of Honey Chocolate Sauce over each pear dish. Refrigerate until cool.

Serves 2

mom's applesauce and toast

My mother taught me this comfort food combination. The applesauce is simple to make and guaranteed to keep the roses in those little cheeks. Make sure to serve it warm.

4 large Delicious apples, peeled, cored,
and quartered
1 cinnamon stick
Unsweetened apple juice
Ground cinnamon
Wheat toast

1. Put apple quarters into a medium-size saucepan. Add the cinnamon stick.
2. Pour in enough apple juice to cover the apples and cinnamon stick.
3. Bring to a boil, then reduce heat and simmer for 20 minutes.
4. Remove from heat and pour out about half of the apple juice. Remove and discard the cinnamon stick.
5. Mash the apples with a fork until they have a lumpy consistency.
6. Add the ground cinnamon to taste. Serve warm with wheat toast or as a spread on wheat toast.

Serves 4

honey peach dip

An ideal dip for springtime fun and good for growing bodies too! Peaches are full of beta-carotene, the vitamin responsible for helping to build strong bones, teeth, skin, and healthy eyes.

4 large ripe peaches

¼ cup honey

¼ cup orange juice

4 slices raisin bread, toasted

1. Peel and chop peaches. Mash them with a fork in a medium-size bowl. Add honey and orange juice.
2. Put bowl in the center of a large plate.
3. Cut the toasted bread into strips. Arrange the strips on the plate around bowl. To eat, dip strips into peach mixture.

Serves 4

melon bowl

It's okay to lick the bowl with this dish. Better yet, you can eat the bowl. Kids have fun with this easy-to-make treat that is good for them. Cantaloupe has significant amounts of carotenes, B-complex vitamins, vitamin C, calcium, phosphorus, and potassium. And it helps build strong eyes.

1 ripe cantaloupe
1 cup sliced fresh strawberries
1 cup frozen vanilla nonfat yogurt
2 whole strawberries

1. Cut cantaloupe in half.
2. Mix sliced strawberries and yogurt together.
3. Spoon half of the mixture into each cantaloupe half. Top each half with a strawberry and a spoon.

Serves 2

strawberry pie

Fresh fruit pies are the best because the vitamins are not baked away. The no-sugar jam in this recipe enhances the sweet combination of strawberries and honey. For an extra-special treat, serve the pie with Mama's Whipped Cream.

1 10-ounce jar no-sugar-added strawberry jam
¼ cup honey
2 cups sliced fresh strawberries
1 baked 9-inch pie shell
Mama's Whipped Cream (page 57), optional

1. Mix jam and honey together. Add strawberries and stir until well coated.
2. Pour strawberry mixture into baked pie shell. Serve, topped with Mama's Whipped Cream if you wish. Be sure to refrigerate any leftovers.

Serves 8

fruit kabobs

Arranging fruit on a stick encourages children to be creative with their favorite fruits. Then try the kabob dipped in Orangey Sauce. Delicious! Please make sure that any small child is well supervised while handling wooden kabob sticks.

Fresh fruit
Wooden kabob sticks
Orangey Sauce (page 58), optional

1. Cut fruit into 1-inch pieces. Any of your favorite fruits will work.
2. Alternate pieces of fruit to make a colorful display on each stick. Children think it's fun to dip the fruit, one piece at a time, into the Orangey Sauce.

frozen favorites

My sons used to love icy treats, but on
a hot summer day you don't have to
be a kid to enjoy a frozen treat.

berry honey cones

It's much more fun to prepare these cones together at home than to buy the less-than-healthy version at the store. The warm honey sauce tastes like it was drizzled from nectar heaven.

1 cup frozen vanilla nonfat yogurt
¼ cup minced blueberries
½ cup favorite granola
4 plain ice cream cones
4 teaspoons warm Honey Sauce (recipe follows)

1. Mix yogurt, blueberries, and granola together in a medium-size bowl. Put mixture in freezer.
2. When the mixture has frozen, remove it from the freezer and scoop it into ice cream cones. Drizzle each cone with a teaspoon of warm Honey Sauce.

honey sauce

¼ teaspoon vanilla extract
¼ cup honey

Combine vanilla and honey in a microwave-safe bowl. Heat in microwave oven on high for 1 minute. Stir again to thoroughly mix.

Serves 4

raspberry creamy pops

Plan ahead for a hot summer afternoon by making these frozen pops in the morning.

> 1½ cups ripe raspberries or a 12-ounce bag
>   unsweetened frozen berries
> ½ cup vanilla nonfat yogurt
> 6 3-ounce paper cups
> 6 popsicle sticks

1. Put berries in blender. Whip until slightly chunky. Stir in yogurt to combine well.
2. Pour this thick liquid evenly into six paper cups. Put a popsicle stick into each cup and freeze until hard.

Serves 6

ᴜnchy lemon pie

ᴊu no longer need to hesitate when your youngster asks for a piece of pie. The ingredients in this pie are good for a growing body and taste terrific with every bite.

2 cups crushed granola
2 tablespoons light margarine, melted
2 cups nonfat lemon frozen yogurt, softened
2 cups crushed cornflakes

1. Mix granola and margarine together. Spread half into the bottom of an 8-inch pie plate. Put in freezer for 15 minutes.
2. Combine yogurt and cornflakes. Spread on top of the cold crust.
3. Cover with remaining granola mixture to form the top crust. Put back in freezer for 1 hour.

Serves 8

coconut cones

My sons used to love to help make foods to freeze. I loved watching their faces light up as we removed the finished product from the freezer. Dipping these cones in coconut or some other natural topping provided that final touch that the kids loved licking off.

½ cup chopped strawberries

½ cup chopped walnuts

1 cup frozen strawberry nonfat yogurt

4 plain cones

¼ cup flaked coconut

1. Mix strawberries and walnuts into frozen yogurt until evenly distributed. Put back into freezer for a half hour.

2. Scoop into cones, dip into flaked coconut, and serve.

Serves 4

cocoa freeze

I hope you have some leftover Honey-Kissed Hot Chocolate, because this dessert is surprisingly fabulous. It is perfect for a lazy afternoon at home because you need to be near the freezer. You and your children can take turns stirring the ice crystals. Trust me, you will love this one!

Any amount of Honey-Kissed Hot Chocolate
(page 25)

1. Pour the chocolate drink into an 8-inch cake pan. Put in refrigerator for about 1 hour. Transfer to the freezer for 30 minutes.

2. Remove pan from freezer. Mix frozen chocolate with a fork, breaking up the ice crystals. Freeze for another 15 minutes, then break up the ice crystals again.

3. Freeze for another 15 minutes, then break up crystals. Do this one more time, then serve immediately, topped with nuts and drizzled with honey if desired.

creamy juice pops

So easy and so savory. Any juice will do. Why not mix a few colorful juices together and see what happens?

1½ cups juice, any favorite flavor
12 tablespoons low-fat milk
6 3-ounce paper cups
6 popsicle sticks

1. Fill the paper cups with half of the juice and freeze for about an hour.
2. Pour 2 tablespoons of milk into each cup and freeze for 30 minutes more.
3. Top with remaining juice, insert sticks in the middle of cups, and freeze until hard.

Makes 6 pops

hot fudge sundaes

This is a lower-calorie and lower-fat version of an American favorite, but it's still loved by kids and grown-ups alike.

Nonfat frozen yogurt, any flavor
Banana slices
Hot Fudge Sauce (recipe follows)
Chopped nuts
Mama's Whipped Cream (page 00)

Get all your sundae ingredients ready. Then prepare the sauce.

hot fudge sauce

2 squares (2 ounces) semisweet chocolate
  (or substitute unsweetened carob chips)
3 tablespoons light margarine
1/4 teaspoon vanilla extract
1/2 cup honey

1. Melt chocolate and margarine in microwave oven for 1 minute on high. Stir in vanilla and honey.
2. Serve the sauce warm over nonfat frozen yogurt, sliced banana, and chopped nuts. Top with Mama's Whipped Cream.

Serves 4

melon icy

What a creative way to get your daily serving of fruit. You may be tempted to drink this treat, but use a spoon to enjoy every tasty bite.

1 cantaloupe, cut into small cubes and frozen
½ cup orange juice

1. Peel cantaloupe. Cut it into small cubes. Freeze in a covered container for 2 hours.
2. Put cantaloupe cubes and orange juice in blender and mix until smooth. Pour into dessert cups and serve.

Serves 2 to 4

pineapple pops

This is another example of vitamin C on a stick. You may want to double this recipe because these leave your freezer fast.

>1 cup unsweetened pineapple juice
>1 cup finely chopped and drained fresh or canned unsweetened pineapple
>6 3-ounce paper cups
>6 popsicle sticks

1. Mix together pineapple juice and pineapple. Pour into the 6 paper cups. Freeze for about 30 minutes.

2. Remove from freezer. Place a popsicle stick in the middle of each cup and freeze until hard, about 1 hour.

Makes 6 pops

Silly Sandwiches

These tasty sandwich concoctions are a far cry from a typical bland sandwich. They are nutritious, fun to make, and can be enjoyed within minutes.

cheese fruit roll-ups

Here's a new way to liven up a tortilla—spread it with flavored cream cheese and perk it up with dried fruits and nuts. For an added treat, try these with Orangey Sauce.

 1/2 cup light cream cheese
 1/4 cup honey
 1/2 teaspoon ground cinnamon
 1/2 cup chopped raisins, dates, or any
   favorite dried fruit
 1/4 cup packaged nut topping
 4 wheat tortillas
 Orangey Sauce (page 58), optional

1. Stir together cream cheese, honey, cinnamon, dried fruit, and nut topping until smooth.

2. Divide mixture into 4 separate parts. Place each part on a tortilla. Roll up and slice into individual pieces.

3. If you wish, arrange the pieces on a plate, surrounding a bowl of Orangey Sauce.

Serves 4

eggy jam sandwiches

Most kids like French toast, so this is a great way to give them some protein while they are eating a treat.

4 eggs

¼ cup low-fat milk

½ teaspoon vanilla extract or pure maple syrup

1 teaspoon ground cinnamon

6 tablespoons light margarine

4 wheat English muffins, cut in halves

4 ounces light cream cheese

½ cup no-sugar-added boysenberry jam

1. In a medium-size bowl, mix eggs, milk, vanilla or maple syrup, and cinnamon until smooth.
2. Melt margarine in large skillet over medium heat.
3. Dip each muffin half in egg mixture and place in skillet. Cook until lightly browned on both sides.
4. Remove each muffin half and put them on a large plate. Spread 4 halves with cream cheese and the other 4 halves with the jam. Put each half with jam on top of the half with the cream cheese.

Serves 4

banana sandwich squares

My sons love peanut butter and banana sandwiches to this day. These squares offer the same flavor and nutrition but with a twist. Serve them warm and they will melt in your mouth.

> 2 ripe bananas, mashed
> 2 tablespoons honey
> ½ teaspoon vanilla extract
> ½ cup chunky low-fat peanut butter
> 6 pieces wheat bread
> Sprinkle of ground cinnamon

1. Preheat oven to 400° F.
2. Mix bananas, honey, vanilla, and peanut butter together until smooth.
3. Spread half of mixture on 2 pieces of the wheat bread. Place 2 more pieces of the bread on top to make 2 sandwiches.
4. Spread remaining mixture on top of sandwiches. Top this with the last 2 pieces of bread, making 2 triple-decker sandwiches.
5. Cut each sandwich into quarters and place onto an ungreased cookie sheet.
6. Sprinkle ground cinnamon lightly onto the sandwich squares and bake for 10 minutes. Serve warm.

Makes 8 squares

bagel smiley faces

Guaranteed to bring smiles and giggles as your little ones create silly faces that they can gobble up afterward.

6 wheat or favorite bagels, cut in half
8 ounces light cream cheese
1 small package trail mix

1. Toast bagels.

2. Spread them with cream cheese. Let the children make faces on the bagels with the different pieces of the trail mix.

Serves 6

cashew butter tamales

I like this recipe because kids just love to roll things up. The delicious ingredients are an all-time favorite, and they're full of protein too! Cashews are also very high in healthy fats, vitamin E, fiber, iron, and calcium.

¼ cup raisins

4 tablespoons cashew or peanut butter

4 tablespoons honey

⅛ teaspoon ground cinnamon

4 wheat tortillas

1. Combine raisins, cashew or peanut butter, honey, and cinnamon. Spread on tortillas. Roll up and cut into bite-size pieces.
2. Place in microwave on high for 30 seconds.

Serves 4

nutty raisin sandwiches

Great party sandwiches! Kids will delight in the different and unique shapes they can create, and they will enjoy them much more because they designed them together.

1½ cups light cream cheese

½ cup raisins

½ cup chopped almonds or favorite nuts

¼ teaspoon ground cinnamon

¼ cup pure maple syrup

12 slices raisin bread

1. Combine cream cheese, raisins, and nuts. Add cinnamon and maple syrup and stir well.

2. Spread 6 pieces of the bread with cream cheese mixture. Top with the remaining bread.

3. Cut sandwiches into quarters or use a cookie cutter to make different shapes.

Serves 6

Slurpy Sauces

These sauces are rich, creamy, and just plain dreamy. No one would ever guess they're full of nutritious ingredients.

honey chocolate sauce

Why settle for store-bought chocolate sauce when you can make it so easily at home? This sauce tastes wonderful and does not leave you with that sweet-sugary aftertaste. It also makes a super icing for your favorite cake. Your children will be begging to lick the bowl. And you won't have to worry about them, because moderate amounts of dark chocolate offer high concentrations of heart-healthy flavonoids. The unsaturated fatty acids found in cocoa butter can actually decrease LDL, or bad cholesterol, according to a study published in the February 2003 issue of the *Journal of the American Dietetic Association*.

> 4 squares (4 ounces) semisweet chocolate
> ¼ cup honey
> ⅓ cup light margarine

1. Melt chocolate and honey in microwave oven on high for 1 minute. Add margarine and stir until smooth.
2. Cool for about a half hour if you plan to use it for cake icing.
3. Store leftover portions in the refrigerator and microwave for 30 seconds to reheat.

Variation: This sauce can be prepared the same way with 4 tablespoons unsweetened carob chips, 4 tablespoons honey, and 2 tablespoons margarine.

Serves 4

mama's whipped cream

No more high-cholesterol, high-fat whipped cream. This whipped cream is low in fat and has no refined sugar, so it's better for you. But it still has a great flavor and dresses up any dessert.

1 12-ounce can evaporated skim milk
½ teaspoon vanilla extract
3 tablespoons pure maple syrup

1. One hour before you want to serve your dessert, put the can of milk in the refrigerator. Also put a large stainless steel bowl and the beaters from an electric mixer into the freezer.

2. Just before serving, pour milk into the chilled bowl. Add vanilla extract and maple syrup. Beat with the chilled beaters at high speed until peaks form. Serve immediately.

Serves 4

orangey sauce

Anyone who likes orange juice and vanilla yogurt will love this simple sauce. Spoon it over any dessert you like or use it as a dip. The orange taste complements most desserts perfectly and is full of vitamin C and protein.

> 2 tablespoons concentrated frozen orange juice, mashed
> ⅛ teaspoon ground cinnamon
> 2 cups vanilla nonfat yogurt

Mix all three ingredients together and chill until ready to serve. Leftover portions must be refrigerated.

Serves 4

lemon cream-cheese sauce

This light and lemony sauce, which doubles as an icing, is quick to make and excellent with many dessert treats. The distinctive flavor of fresh lemon juice adds zing to the light cream cheese, making it a sensational way to complement any baked goodie.

1 cup light cream cheese
½ cup honey
1 tablespoon lemon juice

Mix all three ingredients together until smooth. Spread on a cake for icing or put in a bowl for a sauce. Leftovers or iced cakes must be stored in the refrigerator.

Serves 4

easy peanut butter sauce

This savory sauce almost needs no explanation. It may be simple but it is the stuff dreams are made of. I could put it on everything. It's great spooned over low-fat ice cream, as a dip for sliced fruit, or between low-fat graham crackers. Eat slowly to enjoy the full flavor.

1/4 cup low-fat creamy peanut butter

1/2 cup honey

1/4 teaspoon ground cinnamon

Mix all three ingredients until smooth. Serve right away or store in the refrigerator. Microwave for 30 seconds to warm it up before serving.

Serves 4

index

j

Jam, Sandwiches, Eggy, 49

k

Kabobs, Fruit, 36

l

Lemon
    Cream-Cheese Sauce, 59
    Pie, Munchy, 40
Lemonade, Berry Good, 24

m

Macaroon Muffins, 14
Mama's Whipped Cream, 57
    in Fruity Graham Parfait, 30
    in Hot Fudge Sundaes, 44
    with Maple Cake, 2
    with Strawberry Pie, 35
Maple
    Cake, 2
    Chips, 10
Melon
    Bowl, 34
    Icy, 45
Mom's Applesauce and Toast, 32
Muffins
    Macaroon, 14
    Spicy Oat, 13
Munchy Lemon Pie, 40

n

Nutty Raisin Sandwiches, 53

o

oat(s)
    Muffins, Spicy, 13
    Balls, Peanut Butter, 18
    in Strawberry Jam Bars, 15
Orangey Sauce, 58
    with Cheese Fruit Roll-Ups, 48
    with Fruit Kabobs, 36

p

peach
    Dip, Honey, 33
    Enchiladas, 8
peanut(s)
    in Honey Nut Corn, 3
    in Pea-Nutty Squares, 21
peanut butter
    in Banana Sandwich Squares, 50
    Oat Balls, 18
    in Pea-Nutty Squares, 21
    Sauce, Easy, 60
    Tamales, 52
Pear Sundae, Coolest, 31
pie
    Munchy Lemon, 40
    Strawberry, 35
Pineapple Pops, 46
popcorn
    in Honey Nut Corn, 3

about
the author

Julie Whittingham lives in Apple Valley, California, where she is a wife and a mother of three grown sons who still enjoy her "junkless" baked treats. She attained a bachelor's degree in nutrition from Clayton College and is pursuing her master's and Ph.D. degrees with an eye toward teaching nutrition seminars at colleges and health organizations. Julie is a member of the Coalition for Natural Health, a former manager of two health food stores, and the owner of a convention management company.